Low Carb Diet

Low Carb Diet Plan For Fat Loss For Life! Fast Acting Low Carb Diet To Lose Weight As Soon As Tomorrow!

I0428325

Sarah Brooks

STOP!!! Before you read any further....Would you like to know the Secrets of Body Transformation?

If your answer is yes, then you are not alone. Thousands of people are looking for the secret to rapidly burn body fat, keep the weight off, become healthier, and truly transform their body and life for good.

If you have been searching for these answers without much luck, you are in the right place!

Not only will you gain incredible insight in this book, but because I want to make sure to give you as much value as possible, right now for a limited time you can get full **100% FREE access to a VIP bonus EBook** entitled **THE 7 KEYS TO BODY TRANSFORMATION!**

Just Go Here For Free Instant Access:

www.liveFitVIP.com

Legal Notice

Disclaimer Notice

Table Of Contents

Introduction

I want to thank you and congratulate you for purchasing the book, *"Low Carb Diet: Low Carb Diet Plan For Fat Loss For Life! Fast Acting Low Carb Diet To Lose Weight As Soon As Tomorrow!"*.

This book contains proven steps and strategies on how to get rid of excess weight fast!

So you have found yourself in the position of procrastination. You needed to start dieting months ago to get ready for that special event, or just to get ready to go to the beach or pool this year. Don't dismay you are not alone or too late. There are many proven strategies that can help you lose those extra pounds.

If you need to lose 10 lbs fast, drop a few inches to fit into that dress or maybe to fit into those favorite pants once again, then this book is exactly what you need. It will provide you with all the latest techniques and strategies to give you the surefire way to accomplish your desires in record time.

Don't wait any longer to have the body and health you have been missing out on. Many people wait for a perfect time to get in shape, lose a few pounds, and feel better about themselves, only to lose precious years in the process. The problem is that many times there isn't a perfect time to do anything in our lives.

The perfect time is NOW. If you really want something, there is no such thing as the wrong timing. Just take action now and you will soon be on your way to a much happier life.

Thanks again for purchasing this book, I hope you enjoy it!

Chapter 1: Faster Low Carb Weight Loss Strategies

One of the most common physical problems in our modern world is people gaining unwanted fat in problem areas of their body's. The easy availability of cheap fast food and other unhealthy processed food have caused people to lose control of their diet. After looking in the mirror and realizing how much they have gained, people often are left with feelings of sadness, discouragement, and wondering if their long term health is at risk.

The great Tony Robbins says that we need to see our problems as they are, but not worse than they are. So let us take his advice and realize all we need to do is change a few things in our diet, exercise program, and begin living a healthier lifestyle to fix our seemingly large problems, that in reality are not that hard to fix! So let's not overcomplicate them.

Slimming down does not necessarily mean you have to starve yourself. Provided the right diet and a proper exercise plan, it is not impossible to lose 10 pounds fast. So what does it exactly take to slim down fast enough? Below are some of the most important things you should keep in mind:

- Make complex carbs 30 percent of you calorie consumption

- Make protein 50 percent of your calorie intake

- Make healthy fats 20 percent of the total calories you eat

Avoid the common weight loss mistakes.

When it comes to losing the extra pounds, it is not only important that you learn the things you should be doing. It is equally crucial that you figure out the wrong things you may still be doing. A lot of people do weight loss mistakes without even knowing it. Little do they know what they think can slim them down are actually obstacles to their weight loss goals.

For instance, skipping meals is one of the most common practices. The plain truth is that it is an unhealthy practice. Some people also avoid dairy products altogether. But the fact is calcium contained in dairy products is helpful in burning calories and fat.

Water should not be avoided when dieting. Water can not only burn fat, it also helps the body get rid of toxins. Ice cold water for instance is very good because the body is forced to burn additional calories and fat to make sure the water you drink is properly heated to match your body temperature. You are also more than welcome to dose up on coconut water, fat free milk and other slimming drinks such as green tea, vegetable juice and yogurt based smoothies.

Stick to a healthy diet plan.

You have plenty of food options to include in your diet. The safest bet always includes raw fruits and vegetables. These healthy foods work not only to slim you down but also promote your overall health. These foods also give you energy to perform slimming exercises which can only increase the amount of weight loss.

Sufficient amount of fruits and vegetables included regularly in your daily meals, ensures that you are getting enough fiber from your diet. Fibers are known to be good for digestion and assist in gradual weight loss. Fruits are a little tricky because they do have a higher sugar content, so you will want to make sure you get a serving or two, but also make sure that they don't push you over the edge in the way of your low-carb diet guidelines.

Vegetables on the other hand, are pretty hard to eat too many of, especially the green kind. Think spinach leaves, broccoli, kale, cucumbers, zucchini squash, etc...When you veer off into the colored ones like carrots just make sure you know what is in them, because carrots for instance actually have quite a bit of sugar! This doesn't mean they can't be eaten or that they shouldn't be, it just means moderation is probably a good idea.

Make time for exercise.

Dieting alone will not suffice. Cardiovascular exercises are recommended for overall weight loss. But there are targeted forms of workout too. Know your goal and implement the right type of exercise including the proper equipments for best results.

People tend to avoid exercise thinking that a strict low-carb diet alone can help them get slim. Although true to some extent, it is very difficult to maintain proper weight loss without engaging in suitable exercises from time to time. Doing even light exercises is also effective if done correctly.

Why low-carb diet?

The advantage of a low carb diet over a low calorie diet is that a low-carb diet does not mean eating less food. It just means consuming less carbohydrates and sugar. Even foods having good quantities of fats are acceptable in a low carbohydrate diet plan, and in fact you should eat more healthy fats on a low carb diet to make sure you get the proper amount of calories - but I must stress this - fats add up quick! Be careful, a small handful of nuts, or half an avocado has a lot more calories than you think!

Low carb diets are known to help lose weight and also control blood-sugar level altogether without starving oneself.

The reason low-calorie diet is more popular is that, people think it shows faster and better results. But it also requires plenty of exercise for quick fat loss. Many people think they do not have adequate time for such routines. But I promise you there is time, it doesn't matter how many hours you work, or what your schedule, if you don't make time for your health, it will make time for you! And then it will be an emergency instead of a want.

Many of the world's leading physicians suggest low carb diet to their clients and get better results.

Although the main purpose of this type of diet is to lower carbohydrate intake, it is also important to know that long term deprivation of carbs in your body could damage your metabolism and decreases your fat burning capacity. So it is suggested that a limited but sufficient amount of carbohydrate intake is necessary daily. Also, this is why it is very important to have a higher carb day about one day a week, often called a cheat meal or day. When you do this you must obstain from over eating, this is not a high calorie day, just a high carb day, so this means that when you increase you carbs, you must lower your fats substantially to stay within your calorie range.

It is observed that low-carb diets also show similar outcomes as compared to low-calorie diet, with much less stress on our body. But you still have to manage your diet properly and adjust your eating and drinking habits accordingly.

Keep yourself away from stress. Being stressed gets your body in a state with elevated levels of stress related hormones. Increased stress actually increases your cravings for unhealthier food. This is not good for your low carb diet. If you are unsure of how this can be accomplished, I recommend checking out a book on meditation.

This all means you have to be ready to make changes on your lifestyle. A few sacrifices and compromises are called for here and there, but you know it is worth it when you start to get in a better shape.

Chapter 2: Top Foods For Rapid Fat Loss

Just as the wrong type of food is the reason for gaining those extra pounds of fat, the right type of food will get you slimmed down if taken appropriately, in the proper amounts. Watchful food intake helps you to maintain your body's carbohydrate and sugar levels, keeping you healthy.

A lot of people are under the impression that they have to eat less to weigh less. However, when you eat the right foods, eating more can also lead to weighing less. You just have to find the right foods to indulge in.

This is where a low carb diet is vital. Eating more foods which contain very low carbohydrates actually is a way to fast weight loss. The result of a low carb diet can be similar to a low-calorie diet, with the difference being that you won't need to eat less or stay hungry. When I say less, I don't necessarily mean less calories. I am more focused on the volume of food that goes into your body, Just stop and think about it for a second. A Serving of bread has roughly 100 calories, whereas a serving of spinach leaves has about 15 calories. You can do the math, but at the end of the day, you don't have to feel hungry.

The following is a list of foods that can help boost calorie burning and control your cravings. If you want to slim down fast, you may want to start rearranging your diet and get on with these "slimming" foods.

Eggs

If you happen to have a bagel for breakfast, it will be a good idea to stop. Instead, try eggs. They are filled with protein. Eating eggs can make you feel satisfied for a longer period of time, at least longer than what bagel can achieve. Eggs also contain very low amount of carbohydrates, thus are a good addition to your low carb diet.

According to a multicenter study involving 30 women who were either overweight or obese, those who ate two scrambled eggs plus two slices of toast and a fruit spread actually ate less for the next 36 hours as compared to the women who had bagel for breakfast although it contains the same amount of calories. Another good thing about eggs is their protein content. Protein can actually help prevent fluctuations in the blood sugar level which in turn, help control food cravings.

Salad

Go for the big, low calorie salad with the absence of creamy dressing. In a study conducted by the Penn State University involving 42 women, the subjects who consumed salad ate 12 percent less pasta when they were served with one. It did not matter that they were told they could have as much as they wanted. So, have as much salad as you want.

It will actually help you slim down. In fact, eating salad can increase levels of folic acid, vitamins C and E, carotenoids and lycopene according to the Journal of the American Dietetic Association. All these nutrients are known disease fighters. So, not only do you slim down, salad can also help strengthen your body's defenses.

Beans

Cholecystokinin is a digestive hormone known to help suppress the appetite. And beans are a good source of this natural appetite suppressant according to the University of California at Davis. Moreover, beans can regulate the body's blood sugar levels which allow the body to control hunger. Consuming high fiber beans can also decrease cholesterol levels.

Green Tea

Green tea does contain some amount of caffeine. But that is not exactly what makes it slimming down agent. What is notable about green tea is its catechins content. It is an antioxidant that boosts the fat burning process and speed up the body's metabolic rate.

In a Japanese study involving 35 men, those who consumed one bottle of oolong tea which contains a mixture of green tea not only lost weight. Their metabolism improved and they experienced a significant decrease in their body mass index. It also helped reduce their LDL cholesterol level.

Lean Beef

If you are aiming to slim down but at the same time, maintain calorie burning muscle then you should get a dose of the amino acid leucine. It is found in rich protein sources such as fish, meat and dairy products.

In a study conducted by the University of Illinois at Urbana-Champaign, 24 overweight 50 something women were fed around 9 to 10 ounces of beef daily. This is equivalent to about 1,700 calories. The women lost more weight, shed more fat but lost less muscle mass.

This is compared to the participants who consumed the same amount of calorie diet but with less protein. It is also important to note that the women who consumed lean beef experienced lesser hunger pangs.

Grapefruit

According to a 2006 study from the Nutrition and Metabolic Research Center, drinking one serving of grapefruit juice thrice a day or consuming half a whole grapefruit can help individuals lose over 3 pounds over the course of 12 weeks. This is what 91 obese individuals had experienced during the study. The secret lies with the phytochemical content of grapefruit. It is found to help decrease insulin levels. This is the process responsible for the conversion of calories into energy, preventing conversion to flab.

Soup

Even a cup of chicken soup can leave you feeling satisfied. That is according to a study from the Purdue University. According to the results of the research, a cup of soup is satisfying as the brain perceives it to be.

Pears

Pears contain more fiber according to the calculation from the U.S. Food and Drug Administration. This fruit at a medium size contains about six grams of

fiber. It is equipped with pectin fiber which can reduce blood sugar levels. Otherwise, it may lead to more bouts of hunger.

By reducing your blood sugar levels, a pear can effectively help you avoid snacking in between meals. The results from a Brazilian study involving overweight women showed that those who consumed three pieces of small pears a day for 12 weeks lost more weight than those who snacked on oat cookies.

Cinnamon

If you are experiencing a mid afternoon sugar slump, take oatmeal with cinnamon sprinkled over it. The U.S. Department of Agriculture conducted a research and found out that cinnamon has the ability to regulate insulin spike after meals. That can make you feel rather hungry. A quarter teaspoon of cinnamon does not only help reduce blood sugar. It can also lower triglyceride and cholesterol levels especially in individuals who suffer from type 2 diabetes.

Olive Oil

When you reach mid age, it is much easier to gain extra pounds and much more challenging to lose them. But monounsaturated fat such as extra virgin olive oil can help you burn calories. Results from an Australian study involving 12 postmenopausal women proved that olive oil can help boost metabolism. You can add it to salad dressings, bread dips or even to oatmeal. Make sure you use extra virgin olive oil to sauté your vegetables too.

Nuts

A handful of nuts may amount to 165 calories and that is enough to convince you to stay away. But according to research studies, snacking on nuts can actually make you slimmer. A research from the Purdue University proves that 500 calories of nuts added to a regular diet can help individuals eat less in the subsequent meals. The study that involved normal weight people also showed that snacking on peanuts can also increase resting metabolic rate by as much as 11 percent. This allowed the participants to burn more amount of calories even during their resting time. Nuts that are rich in omega-3 fatty acids such as walnuts are also helpful to your overall health. Whole pecans can help prevent heart disease too.

Vinegar

How does bread dipped in vinegar sound? A Swedish study found that the acetic acid content of vinegar has the ability to inhibit the passage of food to the small intestines from the stomach. This means you can stay full for longer. Vinegar also has the ability to stop sudden increases in blood sugar especially after eating cookies, crackers and white bread.

High Fiber Cereal

The University of Minnesota in Minneapolis and the VA Medical Center conducted an interesting research where the researchers fed participants five cereals before taking them to the buffet table. Among the 14 volunteers, those that consumed cereal with the highest fiber content ate the least from the smorgasbord.

That being said, this is a little tricky and if you want to do cereal you really must do your homework on how many carbs are in them, also don't forget the carbs in the milk. At the end of the day I shy away from cereal and stick to eggs, turkey bacon, and spinach leaves for my breakfast - and I freaking love it!

Tofu

A study was conducted at the Louisiana State University involving 42 overweight women. Some of the participants were served with a chicken appetizer and others were fed tofu appetizer. Those who had tofu ate less during the meal. The lesson learned here is that although tofu may seem too light, it is proved to be an appetite-quashing protein.

Hot Red Pepper

The capsaicin content of hot red pepper and other spices can help suppress the appetite. If you want to lose weight fast, you must make it a point to eat a bowl of hot red pepper regularly. You can mix it to omelet or other meals. Just like the 13 women that participated in a Japanese research study, you will consume less food that you normally would in succeeding meals when you consume breakfast with red pepper as an ingredient.

Vegetables such as broccoli, kale, cabbage and the like are also helpful in your weight loss goals. The point here is you do not have to feel deprived in an effort to slim down. There are plenty of good foods that can help you lose weight fast but at the same time promote good health. The key is to distinguish those that are good from those that are bad for you.

All the food and food categories mentioned above are proven to be effective in a low carb diet bringing about favorable changes in your metabolic system. They need to be eaten on regular basis with proper diet management. It is to be remembered that even though necessary, these food items need to be taken in controlled quantities.

One thing to be kept in mind is that you should try your best to stay away from processed foods which are meant to be for low carb diets.. They are tasty and tempting but contain unhealthy preservatives, maltitol and other artificial ingredients.

Lack of sleep and increased stress on your body will make you want to eat more and increase your fatigue levels, thus making you incapable of eating healthy and performing exercises.   So make sure you get as much sleep as possible.

Chapter 3: Recommended Exercise For Getting Lean & Muscular

It is a fact that weight loss results can be achieved by eating less calories and burning more with the help of exercise. The equivalent of one pound is estimated at 3,500 calories. The best way to lose more pounds is to implement repetitive movement.

Many activities supplement the need of exercise for weight loss. Lifting heavy weights, running, jogging and other types of cardio exercises can be done to achieve desired results. Cardiovascular exercises are considered by many the best way to burn body fat faster in lesser time.

Why cardiovascular workout works best for slimming down?

As mentioned, repetitive movements have a slimming effect. And cardiovascular exercise features repetitive movements targeting the major muscles of the body. Working the body out continuously and for an extended period of time can absolutely help you lose weight quickly.

Cardio exercises keep your heart and lungs in a healthy state thus also maintain your endurance level. Cardiovascular exercises with correct low carb diet helps you keep burning calories for a longer period of time, facilitating weight loss. The end result is healthier looking and leaner body with reduced fat levels.

What type of cardio workout should you choose?

In addition to performing a cardiovascular workout, it is also important that you decide on the type to choose. There are plenty of cardio exercises to pick from. It is highly recommended that you choose what you absolutely like doing. This way, you can get easily motivated to finish and follow through your exercise routine. If you work out more then you have better chances of slimming down fast.

For instance, if you like to run then take that. If you own a bike then you may want to go biking. Swimming, rowing, brisk walking and elliptical training will also do. But if you are the social type, you may want to try indoor cycling, cardio dance class or step aerobics. Kickboxing is also a good idea. And you are free to mix and match the classes and your workout sessions to keep it interesting and enjoyable.

How long should you do cardio?

The key to slimming down fast is to work out often and long enough. According to the American College of Sports Medicine, a 60 to 90 minute workout for five days a week can help you achieve the best results. If you cannot afford to spend five days a week in the gym, you can also perform multiple bouts in a single day in order to accumulate the time. The same method will be useful for your weight loss goals too.

While performing the exercises it is of utmost importance that you stay hydrated. Water helps to diminish carbohydrate cravings and also your dietary requirements are met with as the carbs are discarded from your body. Water is the crucial element that supplements the process of fat burning and thus needed to be consumed in essential quantity.

What other ways can get you fast results?

It is also recommended that you perform interval training. Such method will help you further with achieving the best weight loss results. So, try to alternate your routine from fast to slow, back and forth. Do this for the entire duration of the exercise.

Interval training helps the body burn more calories. Also, you should not forget to perform a light warm up. After the workout, you should also perform a light cool down. When you do fast and slow, try it in 1 to 2 ratios. So for instance, when you do fast running for 20 seconds, you should do brisk walking for 40.

This method not only burns more calories, but also keeps them burning for longer period of time. High intensity interval training is really effective as your body starts burning fat faster. A low carbohydrate-moderate fat-high protein diet is suitable for intense training, along with sufficient quantity of water.

Other Recommendations

In addition to cardiovascular workout, you should also perform strength training. This is not only for people who want to build muscle. And this is a method that is not exclusive to guys. The thing is your metabolic rate tends to improve when you lift weights and build muscle. As a result, your metabolic rate receives a boost even while resting. That means your body becomes capable of burning calories even when you are not performing any form of exercise. And that can add to your overall calorie burn for an entire day.

The University of Michigan Health System says when you add one pound of muscle; your body can burn extra 30 or up to 50 calories in one day. For strength training, it is recommended that you perform particular exercises that are meant to target major muscle groups. Such includes shoulder presses, triceps pushdowns, back rows, bench presses, squats and biceps curls.

Another important fact about strength training is that it is helpful in order to maintain a slim body. A person builds good amount of muscle near the abdomen area with proper exercises which prevents the dreaded return of belly fat. That is why weight training is required for long term preservation of a flat stomach. Different low carb diet plans are suited with different exercise regimens and you have to decide which one you need to follow as per the results you desire.

Also you have to regulate your supplement consumption so as to not let it interfere with your diet. Supplements that curb carbohydrate cravings are also available, but should be taken only after consultation with physician.

Carb intake and Workouts

A low carbohydrate diet is essential to keep your sugar level at a healthy level, but carbs can be consumed before or after your workouts. If you take carbs during or after/ before your workouts, it does not have a damaging effect on your sugar level. Instead, it will maintain your carbohydrate level so that you can burn fats during workouts, otherwise long term deprivation from carbohydrates can lower your fat burning capacity. So make sure to indulge in some limited carb rich foods before or after intense workout schedules.

Regular carbohydrate refill

Your metabolism can be affected if you are deprived of carbs and calories for long time. Hence, if you are following a low-carb diet strictly, you should have a big quantity of carbohydrate consumption after every few days to refill your body carb storage. We spoke about this earlier, regarding cheat meals/days. This makes carbs readily available when required during workouts and does not lower your energy levels.

Chapter 4: Ways To A Flatter Abs And A Slimmer Waist

Tummy fat is probably one of the most difficult to get rid of. A slim waist is what every man and woman aims for. And you are right to aspire for one too. A flat tummy does not only make you more physically appealing. It is also much healthier.

A slimmer waist does not always mean lower body weight. Infact less body weight may cause weakness. A slim waist just means no unwanted fat around the tummy. You can eat normally and still have flat abs by controlled carb diet and some workout. Low carbohydrate intake means that you will burn more fat during any workout. You can aim for exercises that target your tummy.

Fat deposited around your waist can actually increase your risks to the most life threatening diseases including hypertension, heart disease and some forms of cancer. People have been getting treated for all the above physical problems since a long time. But the only way such diseases can be avoided is by keeping your body fat to a minimum. In addition to eating the right kind of foods, below is a list of suggested exercises that have been proven to help sculpt your waistline and strengthen your core.

Cardiovascular Workout

Cardio exercises are one of the best ways to slim down your waistline. If you want targeted exercises that eliminate belly fat, you must employ the specific cardio workouts meant for this purpose. Go for those that are focused on the abs.

Among the recommended activities are swimming, running, trail hiking and tennis. These workouts burn body fat and at the same time, work on your abs. Other exercises such as kickboxing and using the rowing machine will be very beneficial in achieving a trimmed waistline too.

Abdominal Crunches

This form of exercise works out the four major muscle groups of the abdomen. In other words, it can flatten and strengthen the ab area. If you want a flatter tummy, you should perform the crossover ad crunches, the ab crunch, the stomach crunch, crisscross and vertical leg ab crunch. You can also increase the intensity of these workouts for better results.

AB Machines

For the oblique, using the Roman and the captain's chair are strongly recommended. The lever seater hip raise crunch machine should be taken advantage of. This machine simulates a reverse curl and crunch workout targeting both the lower and upper abs. Other machines such as the torso twist are also recommended for an oblique focused workout.

Floor Exercises

Although floor exercises provide lesser resistance than ab machines, they are quite useful as well in slimming down the waistline. The American Council on Exercise highly recommends the bicycle exercise. This workout is focused on the oblique and the rectus abdominus.

Other helpful exercise methods include the Pilates and particularly, the crisscross, double leg stretch, teaser and roll up routines can help you sculpt a much leaner abs. If you want to further engage your core muscles, make sure to add the scissor kicks to your routine.

Ball Exercises

The ball is one of the most reliable equipment for core work. If you are working out at home, the American Council on Exercise suggests you do the stability ball crunch. In fact, it is number three on the most effective workouts for the rectus abdominus and number six on working out the oblique. If you want to upgrade your level of difficulty, you can also do the stability ball knee tuck as it enhances abdominal strength.

Doing high intensity cardio workouts 3 to 4 times a week has proven to be very effective. Of course, all these exercises will do no good if you do not control you carbohydrate intakes. The more carbs you eat, the less fats are utilized by the body as fuel.

If you are opting for low intensity workouts, it is just as fine. If you are generally an active person on a daily basis, then doing low intensity exercises like walking, jogging, steps, etc. can give you good results too.

Calories Matter

A low carb diet is effective because it reduces your general appetite and makes you eat lesser calories naturally. But if you still consume excess calories, it will adversely affect your diet. Maintain normal calories per day to reach your daily calorie deficit.

Patience with the diet

It is to be noted that at the early stages of your low carb diet you will notice fast weight loss for a few weeks, but then will gradually slow down. It may seem that there is no more fat loss occurring in the body. This is usually the phase where a person lets his or her patience get the best of them. But the fact is if you trust your diet and stick to it, the weight loss will continue gradually. Always remember to replenish your body's carbohydrate stock at regular intervals to assist burning of fats during cardiovascular and strength workouts.

Chapter 5: Recommended Exercises For Toned Legs And Thighs

If you are aspiring to slim down, you may be after toned legs and thighs too. In addition to a cardio workout, there are specific routines focused on slimming down your legs and thighs as well. If you want shapely results, here is the list of the most suggested exercises for sexier and slimmer legs and thighs.

Squats

To do the squat, stand on your feet in hip width apart. Slowly lower yourself as if you are about to sit in an imaginary chair. Lower yourself until your thighs are positioned parallel to the ground then slowly stand back up and move back to the starting position.

Reverse Lunge

Start on a standing position and let your feet flat against the floor. Put one leg behind and lower your back knee. Press the back leg and slowly return to the starting position. Now, do the other leg with the same number of reps.

Side Lunge

Your feet should be a little wider than hip width distance. Place one foot to your side and extend it as far to the side as you can and at the same time, lower your body to the ground. But you have to make sure to keep the other leg straight. Push off the leg that's bent to move back to the starting position.

Forward Lunge

Begin on a standing position with your feet comfortably flat on the floor. Move one foot in front and extend it as far as you can. Then, slowly drop your back knee to the ground. Press off the back leg and return to the standing position.

Curtsy Lunge

In a standing position, place your feet at a hip width distance. Place one leg behind. Cross it behind your front leg. This should prompt both knees toward the ground. Push off the back knee and return to the original position.

Abduction

Lie on your side. Lift the top leg slowly and lower it down. To make this exercise more challenging, you may want to wear ankle weights or place a dumbbell on the leg outside the knee.

Adduction

Lie on the ground on your side. Cross the top leg over to the bottom leg. Lift the bottom leg while keeping the torso from rocking backward. Make sure to perform the same number of reps on the other leg.

Walking Lunges

Stand straight and place your hands on the hips. Step one foot forward and drop the back knee to the ground. Move back to the starting position and try the exercise using the other foot.

Wall Sit

Stand straight with your feet at a hip width distance. Rest your back against the wall. Now, walk your feet out a few inches from the wall and lower your body toward the ground. Lower yourself until your thighs become parallel to the ground. Hold the position and count 30 to 60. Then return to the initial position.

You can also see great results with jump squats, speed walking and dancing. Other excellent thigh slimming exercises for fast results include running, kickboxing, cycling and jump roping.

Another recommended exercise that can work excellently for toned legs and inner thighs is the duck squat. To increase the intensity of this exercise, you can perform it using either a kettle ball or a dumbbell. The American Heart Association recommends that you allot at least 30 minutes of your time doing these exercises. That should give you better results.

Carbs and lower body

Lower body workouts like leg and thigh exercises require a lot of energy and stamina. It is not easy to lift these body parts when first venturing into low carb dieting. If your body is not accustomed to using fats as fuel it can be difficult, but once you get used to a cow carbohydrate diet your body will slowly shift towards fats as a primary source of fuel. So be a little patient and keep in mind your workouts will improve.

Again, as mentioned before, consume the majority of your daily your carbs around your workout schedule so as to maintain your energy level and also keep your blood-sugar levels in check.

Managing the restrictions and consumption of carbohydrates in your diet along with suitable, essential exercises, is what a low carb diet is all about.

Conclusion

Thank you again for purchasing this book about fat loss for life through low carb dieting! I am extremely excited to pass this information along to you, and I am so happy that you now have read and can hopefully implement these strategies going forward.

I hope this book was able to help you to gain some insight on how you can accomplish your goals and lose those extra pounds. Also, if you know of anyone else that could benefit from the information presented here please alert them of this book.

The next step is to get started is to get started using the techniques you have learned in this book to live a much happier, healthier and more fulfilling life!

Finally, if you enjoyed this book and feel that it has added meaning to your life in any way, please take the time to share your thoughts and post a review on Amazon. It'd be greatly appreciated!

Thank you and good luck!

Preview Of:

<u>Honey And Natural Remedies</u>

Incredible Ways For Using Honey, Apple Cider Vinegar, Cinnamon, Lemon, And Many More Natural Remedies To Boost Energy And Restore Health!

Introduction

I want to thank you and congratulate you for purchasing the book, *"Honey And Beyond - Incredible Uses For Honey And Your Health"*.

This book contains insight on the amazing and healthy uses of Honey!

In your search for treatments for some common health issues such as a simple abdominal ache or the common cold, you may have encountered expensive, yet ineffective solutions. I truly understand how it feels to spend a lot and end up with basically no benefits from the artificial remedies. This is where honey enters the picture.

In this book I have presented some of the basic uses of honey. Along with these uses are some of the most promising benefits that honey individually can offer you, as well as, uses of honey in concert with other ingredients. Should you decide to use the sweet liquid with some of the other interesting ingredients you can readily find in the kitchen, here is a short teaser of some of the dynamic combinations. In this book you will find honey paired with combining agents such as: nutmeg, cinnamon, apple cider, cane vinegar, and lemon extract.

Hopefully, the information that you can get out of this book can help you come up with natural, affordable, and safe alternatives for some of the most common pressing problems that you have to face, medically or otherwise.

Thanks again for purchasing this book, I hope you enjoy it!

Chapter 1: Pure Honey And Its Uses

Pure honey is one of the most beneficial food items that nature can give you. In fact, people from the past highly valued this food not just because it helped them satiate their hunger, but also because of its medicinal properties. Today honey is used and supplying many benefits that you cannot readily acquire from other raw food sources. This book will let you in on some of the uses that pure honey can bring once you consume or apply it. Because of the plethora of uses and benefits of honey I did not want to overcomplicate this book causing the reader to search with a fine tooth comb for the answers he or she is looking for. So instead of writing it in a story like fashion I wrote it in a much easier format for the reader to find the use they are looking for. As an added benefit to the reader, this will also act as a much easier reference guide in the future. I hope you enjoy some of the amazing benefits and uses as much as I have!

Face Wash

Using the substance as a facial wash is one of the typical applications for pure honey that can bring a lot of benefits to your skin. You simply have to combine warm water with a small drop of honey. Then, you may directly apply the mixture on your face and gently massage it in using circular strokes. You should keep in mind that the strokes should be done upward and outward. After you have conditioned the skin, thoroughly wash the honey off your skin with cool water. Washing off the honey with cool water will also result in helping your face keep its moisture.

Hair Shine

Honey was even used during the ancient times in history to enhance hair luster. To do this, you need to mix a teaspoon of honey to one quart of water, preferably the water should be warm so you can dilute the sweet substance easily. You may directly apply the mixture on your hair and let it soak indefinitely. In case you are wondering, you do not have to rinse off the concoction as you have already diluted it in the first place. Interestingly, the mixture can also help you calm the frizzles down found at the end of your hair strands.

Antimicrobial Substance

Honey can also be useful in cleaning up some fresh wounds and cuts. This sweet substance works in similar fashion as antibiotic creams. Because pure honey is antimicrobial by nature you may directly apply it on your minor burns, cuts, and some scrapes. You may do this using a clean hand or an applicator. After applying the honey you may want cover the wound using sterile gauze or bandages.

Anti-anxiety Agent
Mixing pure honey with some of your favorite tea brews can enhance the calming effect of these warm drinks. Honey can further improve the effects of the drinks as far as anxiety relief is concerned. You may also add this substance to other drinks such as lemon juice and ginger ale. In fact, you may even combine these two latter liquids with tea and honey to make another interesting drink. The ratio of each component will purely depend upon your own preferences.

Bath Essential

If you happen to be a fan of bath oils and salts you may want to consider using honey as an organic substitute. To do this you need to combine three tablespoons of pure honey to bath water. If you want to really go wild you can add in the combining agent - olive oil (around two tablespoons) and you have an interesting twist to your bathing experience! If you use this mixture regularly you will enjoy a conditioned and well-moisturized skin, not to mention a pleasant odor as well.

Precaution

These are just some of the benefits from using honey. If you are unsure about your body's reactions once you apply honey on your skin or ingest the fluid internally you should seek consultation with your physician first. Most likely the doctor will advise you to undergo a series of tests for an allergy to honey, these tests will take around two weeks to complete. For this procedure, you may be temporarily restricted from consuming honey and other types of similar substances. In case the physician discovers that you have some allergic reactions to the sweet substance, you should refrain from consuming honey all together until your doctor says otherwise. If you still want to do so, you may ask your physician to make the necessary adjustments to help you out. The take home here is that if you have any doubt at all whether or not you are allergic or may have an allergic reaction to honey or any other ingredients in this book, it is best to find out for sure by seeking the proper medical advice by a professional.

Thanks for Previewing My Exciting Book On Honey Entitled:

"Honey And Natural Remedies!"

To purchase this book, simply go to the Amazon Kindle store and simply search:

"HONEY AND NATURAL REMEDIES"

Then just scroll down until you see my book. You will know it is mine because you will see my name "Sarah Brooks" underneath the title.

Alternatively, you can visit my author page on Amazon to see this book and other work I have done. Thanks so much, and please don't forget your free bonuses

DON'T LEAVE YET! - CHECK OUT YOUR FREE BONUSES BELOW!

Free Bonus Offer: Get Free Access To The www.LiveFitVIP.com VIP Newsletter!

Once you enter your email address you will immediately get free access to this awesome newsletter!

But wait, right now if you join now for free you will also get free access to the "The 7 Keys To Body Transformation" free EBook!

To claim both your FREE VIP NEWSLETTER MEMBERSHIP and your FREE BONUS eBook on THE 7 KEYS TO BODY TRANSFORMATION!

Just Go To:

www.liveFitVIP.com

www.ingramcontent.com/pod-product-compliance
Lightning Source LLC
Chambersburg PA
CBHW070938290526
45795CB00003B/1069